Piece of Cake

A Pocket Guide Full of Easy Tips and

Tricks For Everyday Weight Loss

KAYLA MOFFETT

Piece of Cake
A Pocket Guide Full of Easy Tips and Tricks for Everyday Weight Loss

www.KaylaWeightLoss.com

ISBN: 0974459992
ISBN-13: 978-0-9744599-9-8

Dedication

To the love of my life, Michael Stevenson. Without your love and support, there is no way this book would have ever been possible. You're amazing, I love you, and I can't wait to marry you!!

Piece of Cake

Acknowledgements

Thank you to my parents Leslie and Cory for teaching me at a young age to work hard for the things that I want.

My brother and sisters Bryan, KaRynn and Karalee for always being there for me.

My original mentor Richard Greenley for showing me how to run a business and stay "motiv8d" when I was only 19.

My best friend Kevin DeBouse for always being an amazing friend and support.

My accountibillibudy Stephanie Ford for being my support throughout my weight loss journey.

My mentors and coaches, who have helped me to lose 70 pounds!

People who I have coached and mentored along the way. I have learned more from you than you think!

All of my amazingly supportive friends and family.

The amazing love of my life Michael, who empowers and changes people's lives everyday, and shows so many people how to go after their dreams.

Table of Contents

Table of Contents

Introduction

I remember the day I stepped on the scale and saw my "scary number" for the FIRST time. I had no clue how I got to that point.

I grew up extremely active in dance and cheer, but once I hit 21, the pounds slowly started to add on.

I didn't feel that I was eating *that* badly, I knew that I wasn't as active as I used to be, but I didn't understand how I could have gained so much weight so quickly.

I immediately went on a very strict hardcore diet. I downloaded a calorie counter app on my phone and changed my lifestyle dramatically overnight.

No more fried foods, no more creamy foods, no dessert, and no alcohol. I started realizing just how awful things like ice cream were for my body, and with my calorie count of 1,200 calories per day (I was starving!). There just wasn't any room for indulging.

After a couple months of this craziness, I found myself hitting a plateau. I had no clue why I couldn't lose a pound! I hadn't even hit the high number of my recommended weight range yet! I was at the gym everyday, I was on an extremely strict diet, and I NEVER cheated. It made <u>no</u> sense.

A couple of weeks later, I decided that it wasn't worth it anymore. I was bored, I missed hanging out with my friends, and I felt ridiculous going on dates and ordering side salads with lemon squirted on it for dressing, and I wanted a cheeseburger and fries *soooo* bad!!

I very quickly returned to all of my bad habits, which was easy since I felt so deprived the last few months. Within one year I gained back all of my weight <u>plus</u> an extra 20 pounds.

I then conceded defeat and decided that I was just meant to be a "big girl" for the rest of my life. I felt there was nothing that I could do about it.

I did what so many other people do, and just blamed it on my genes. I wasn't willing to be on a strict diet for the rest of my life, and surgery wasn't an option. So I learned to just "deal with it."

I sat in that awful place for a few years until my baby sister told me the news that she was getting married, and in just a month and a half. So basically, I had 45 days to lose 70 pounds for the pictures. I did NOT want to be the "big sister" in the pictures that would forever be on her wall.

Now, obviously losing 70 pounds in 45 days isn't possible, but I went into panic mode and started the dreaded diet again. I even remember going to the gym and asking for a one-month membership. They told me no, but I explained how I wasn't trying to get healthy… I just wanted to lose a few pounds for the wedding! They looked at me like I was a nutcase, tried to talk me into taking it seriously, and I ended up settling on the two-month minimum membership plan.

I ended up losing 20 pounds for the wedding, but that week something shifted for me. I started getting good feedback from my friends, family and customers at work, and I started feeling a little better about myself. I decided that I wanted to keep up my weight loss, but I knew that what I was doing wasn't going to work.

Thankfully, my good friend Stephanie talked me into joining Weight Watchers® with her. I remember being really hesitant about it, but I later learned so many great lessons from them.

I learned that you don't need to be on a super-strict diet to lose weight, and that not eating enough food can backfire. (Hence the plateau on my previous attempt.) I learned that "dieting" is hard, but eating healthy is so much easier and will help you maintain your weight loss once you hit your goal. I learned that it's ok to splurge every once in a while, and that having a coach and support system is extremely important.

I lost over 70 pounds that year, and life has been amazing ever since. My confidence has skyrocketed, I'm so much happier, and I'm no longer afraid of the camera. I can cross my legs when I sit down, and I'm comfortable at the beach. I met the love of my life, actually felt worthy of a man like him. And, I've started a new career as a weight loss coach helping other people hit their goals just like I have.

While on my journey, I was constantly searching for and collecting tips and tricks to make my weight loss efforts easier and smoother.

This book is filled with over 400 tips and tricks that may help you with whatever weight loss plan you may be following (even if you're not following one).

Some of the tips may be just what you're looking for, and some may not. But grab a highlighter, mark your favorites, and feel free to add your own ideas to the collection.

Part 1:
The Basics

Losing weight doesn't have to be hard. It's actually fairly easy if you understand the math. Basically the calories your taking in needs to be less than the calories your body is burning.

This doesn't mean that you can survive on next to nothing. If you aren't taking in enough calories, your body can go into starvation mode, and will start clinging to every calorie it can get.

The easiest thing you can do to start losing weight is to make small changes that will have big impacts. Portion control, substitutions, focusing on healthier choices, and moving more will make all the difference in your weight loss efforts.

Practice Portion Control

One of the biggest lessons to learn while losing weight is that portion control is key. Indulging a little bit every once in a while will keep you from going insane. Overindulging is where you get in trouble.

Having a bite of cake will not make you gain weight, however, having a piece of cake every single day, or eating a whole cake may be a different story.

No matter what plan you are on, eventually you will need to learn how to maintain your weight AFTER you've hit your goal. The fact that so many people go on a crash diet then gain the weight back, then crash diet again, and gain the weight back again shows something. Strict diets aren't always the answer. Sometimes it's smarter to take the simple route, and just learn to cut back.

There is no magic wand or pill that will make you thin forever. Even people who have major surgeries often gain the weight back when they don't learn how to stay healthy. You'll need to learn how to become a healthy person in order to stay the weight you want. Portion control is key in this process.

🍰 If you tend to eat too much of a home cooked meal, make it a point to prepare a half-sized recipe to avoid putting seconds on your plate.

🍰 When putting leftovers away, portion them out into single-serving containers to re-heat the perfect portion and avoid overeating.

🍰 Use small salad plates instead of big dinner plates. This will satisfy your mind with a full plate, but will keep you from overdoing it.

🍰 Never eat out of a bag or basket. Always portion out onto a plate or bowl what you plan on eating, and then stop with that portion.

🍰 Share a plate with a friend at a restaurant, or ask the server for a second plate or box that you can divide your food into. If the second plate is too tempting, ask the server to toss it, or you can cover it in salt or sugar so it's inedible.

🍰 Pass on combo meals, and just order your items à la carte. Or be sure that the sides are healthy – not fries, fried rice, or other high calorie foods.

🍰 When going after something sweet, cut a small piece, enough to have just a taste and then savor it.

🍰 Slow down while you eat. Give your brain time to catch up to let you know when it's full. Do your best to stop eating when you feel you are a six on a scale from one to ten.

🍰 Fill up on veggies, fruits and water first before you start into the main course, so you don't take in a giant amount of high calorie foods.

🍰 Make decisions throughout your day and week. Ask yourself, "Would I rather have 'this' item, or is it more important for me to save the calories for 'that' item I've been craving for later?"

🍰 Eat your meals free of distraction. If you're chowing down mindlessly in front of the TV, you will be inclined to eat more than you would if you were eating free of distractions at the kitchen table.

🍰 Learn how to eyeball portion sizes. Three ounces of protein is about the size of a deck of cards. If it's a long thin slice of fish, three ounces would be about the size of a checkbook.

🍰 The size of a baseball is roughly equal to one cup and can be used to determine how much cereal to pour in the morning. This makes half of a baseball about half a cup. This is a good size for rice or pasta for most women working towards losing weight.

🍰 A medium baked potato is about the size of a bar of soap or a computer mouse.

🍰 An ounce of diced cheese is about the size of three dice.

🍰 Two tablespoons is about the size of a Ping-Pong ball. This is a generous amount of almond butter or dressing for your salad.

🍰 Imagine the size of a CD to decide how much deli meat or cheese to put on sandwiches. Each CD size is about one ounce. One ounce of cheese, and three ounces of meat is ideal.

Acknowledge Cravings

Splurging in moderation every once in a while can actually help you in the long run. It will help shock your body back into "lose mode" and it will keep you from going crazy. Once someone tells you that you can't have something, it will just make you want it more.

🍰 Set aside up to a fifth of your caloric intake for something sweet, or whatever you are craving each day. It will help keep you from feeling deprived.

🍰 Most cravings will go away in 20 minutes. Try to hold out, and if you're still craving it, then go for it keeping portion control in mind.

🍰 Decide if you're actually having a craving, or if you're just hungry. Will something healthy do the trick? Or is it really about the craving?

19

🍰 Also decide if it's an emotional craving. Your body doesn't crave cake, your emotions crave cake. Your body may be craving sugar, but usually a piece of fruit will do the trick.

🍰 Pair your craved item with something healthy to help you fill up faster, and to keep you from overdoing it. For instance, go for chocolate with strawberries, or caramel with an apple. Even if you're craving a cheeseburger, pair that with a garden salad or side of fruit.

🍰 Find healthier substitutions for your cravings. If you're craving chocolate, grab a small cup of hot chocolate. One packet of sugar-free hot cocoa is only about 55 calories. It's fewer calories than a candy bar at 220-300 calories, it will take longer to drink, and you'll be able to savor and enjoy it longer.

🍰 If you're craving something fried like french fries or chicken strips, whip up a batch at home in the oven.

🍰 If you're going to splurge, go gourmet. Make it worth it. The bland store bought chocolate chip cookies just aren't worth the calories! And once you have one, and the craving is still there, you'll keep wanting to eat until the craving is handled. Just find something good to take care of the craving from the get-go.

🍰 If you take a bite of something, and it just isn't doing the trick, stop eating it and get something else instead. Stop feeling bad for wasting nasty foods. It's better to waste it in the trash than to waste it in your body.

Fruits and Juices

Any plan that encourages you to eat a lot of fruits and veggies is a plan that I love. Yes fruits are higher in carbs, BUT think about it this way.

1. Bananas: 105 calories, 27 g carbs, 3.1 g fiber, 0.4 g fat, 1.3 g protein
2. 10 hard, salted pretzels: 108 calories, 48 g carbs, 1.8 g fiber, 1.6 g fat, 6 g protein
3. Bottle Bud Light®: 110 calories, 7 g carbs, 0 g fiber, 0 g fat, 1 g protein

All three of these items are very similar in calorie count, but which do you think is best for your body? There is so much more nutrition in a banana, and they have nutrients your body needs.

If you're looking for a snack, and you only have 100 calories to spend, and you pick a piece of fruit over other snacks, you are helping yourself become more healthy.

Many weight loss plans offer "free" fruits and veggies on their plan, meaning you don't have to count the calories when journaling your intake.

This is great, because it encourages you to make smarter choices throughout the day, and helps you get the nutrients that your body needs.

Obviously you don't want to eat a whole watermelon (that's a lot of sugar in one sitting!) but you should never feel guilty about eating fruits, even those higher in calories.

📑 Be cautious with juices, especially with juices that aren't freshly squeezed. If you're interested in juicing, make sure that you drink whole juice instead of extracted juice. Whole juicers work more like a blender, and use the whole fruit versus a juice extractor, which only pulls the waters, sugars, and some of the nutrients, but leaves the pulp and fiber behind.

🍰 The point of eating fruits and veggies is to get good amounts of fiber and other nutrients in your diet.

🍰 You also want to make sure that you drink the juice right after its been juiced. It starts losing nutrients very quickly, so it's best to make a new serving rather than storing extra for later.

🍰 Add as many veggies as you can to your juices. I get that the idea of adding veggies may turn you off a bit, but you don't want a big glass of ONLY fruits. That is way too much sugar, and when it's juiced, your body will absorb the sugar much quicker.

🍰 Avoid juices from the grocery store. They're not fresh, they are full of added sugars, they contain little- to no fiber, and they're not very nutritious. These juices are just as bad as a soda.

🍰 Keep in mind that it takes several servings of fruits and veggies to fill a glass of juice. You don't want to drink several glasses of juice on top of whole meals each day. They can add a lot of calories to your daily intake, and if you're exceeding the recommended amounts for your age and gender, they could do more harm than good.

🍰 Find new ways to enjoy your fruit, like making it your dessert! Slice a banana lengthwise, and top with low-fat frozen yogurt and chopped almonds.

🍰 Campfire bananas are a great alternative to s'mores. Slice a small slit in the banana and stuff a few chocolate chips inside. Close the fruit back up, wrap in foil, and toss it into the campfire for a few minutes.

🍰 Add fruits like peaches, mango and pineapple to homemade salsas for a new tropical twist for your fish.

🍰 You could even grill your fruits. Make a kebab with pineapple, bananas and peaches to grill on low for a few minutes until warm.

🍰 Freeze your fruits for a new texture and taste. They take longer to eat that way, which makes you eat slower.

Veggies

Veggies make the world go 'round. Well… they do when you're losing weight!

One common recommendation when losing weight is to not count the calories of your veggies at all. If you are building a salad, and you're making smart decisions, but you're counting every last calorie for every piece of broccoli that you put on your salad, two things will happen.

1. It will drive you NUTS!!! Those 20 calories aren't going to hurt you; they're only going to help you. And making yourself look up how many calories are in each little veggie will become tedious and frustrating.

2. You'll end up missing out on veggies you would normally eat. If you're close to your daily limit, and you know you're interested in a glass of wine that night, you may pass on a few veggies just to save calories. Not a good idea.

🍰 Eat 'em up! No guilt!! The great thing is that after a short while, you'll start loving veggies even more. You may even start craving them. I know, it may sound crazy, but it's true!

🍰 The only veggies you should be cautious of are the ones that are high in fats and carbs. This includes potatoes, sweet potatoes, yams, avocado, and edamame. These foods aren't bad for you, but you don't want to down a whole avocado with each meal either. Just indulge in small portions, or count the calories of these vegetables.

🍰 Don't reward yourself or your kids for eating vegetables. This creates a mentality that vegetables aren't good, and keeps them from being enjoyed.

🍰 Find ways to sneak veggies into your favorite recipes. There are several substitutions you can use, like spaghetti squash instead of pasta, but there are other ways to healthify your recipes.

🍰 Try adding a bunch of diced veggies into your ground beef or turkey when grilling it for tacos. You end up with half the amount of meat in your meal, and add a whole new flavor! Onions, jalapeños, garlic, peppers, zucchini, eggplant, mushrooms, and corn are delicious with ground meats.

🍰 The same goes for adding veggies to many recipes, including lasagna, meatloaf, scrambled eggs, soups, pastas, and mashed potatoes.

🍰 Find different ways to enjoy your veggies. Munching on raw carrots and celery all day isn't for everyone, so find out what works for you!

🍰 Find new dips to take your vegetables skinny-dipping in! Use hummus, almond butter, Laughing Cow® cheese wedges, or tzatziki sauce instead of ranch dips for a lighter dip full of flavor.

🍰 Add a whole new flavor by drizzling your veggies with balsamic vinegar.

🍰 Keep frozen bags of vegetables in the freezer for times when your fresh veggies start to look a little sad.

🍰 Get a steamer! This is my favorite kitchen appliance. Pour some water in the bottom, add some veggies in the basket, and five minutes later you have a fantastic snack or side dish for your dinner. Be sure to have your veggies pre-prepped and sliced for the week. It makes it so much easier to just throw them into the steamer rather than having to clean, cut and prep them each time.

🍰 Get a juicer! A good one that won't hold back all the pulp and fiber. Use as many veggies as you can, and use a little fruit to sweeten it up.

⬦ Get a griller! Whether it's a BBQ, or even a George Forman Grill™, it adds a whole new flavor to your good ol' faithful veggies. Lay them flat on the grill, put them on a skewer or wrap a bunch in tin foil and use a little olive oil spray (always spray the oil rather than pouring it) and you'll have a batch of delicious grilled veggies for snacks or side dishes.

⬦ Get a deep fryer! *Just kidding!!!* Pass on that one. If you already have it, repurpose it into an herb garden, re-gift it, or just sell it on eBay.

Random Tips and Tricks

Here are a few easy go-to tricks that can help you in your everyday weight loss.

🍰 Eat on a smaller plate. You are able to fill up the plate and mentally feel like you have more food, rather than having a half empty large plate.

🍰 Do your best to fill up half of your plate with fruits and veggies.

🍰 Using chopsticks, a smaller fork, or using your non-dominant hand to eat will help you slow down and eat slower. This will allow your body time to tell your brain that you are full so you don't overeat.

🍰 Slice up your food. You'll feel more satisfied because you feel like you ate more. This goes for chips and anything else. Break them up so you feel like there are more pieces to eat.

🍰 Be well-rounded and make sure to eat from all of the major food groups each day, including dairy and healthy fats.

🍰 Drink a lot of water. Your body often confuses thirst with hunger.

🍰 Be cautious with white foods. That is the color of several high fat and high carb foods with less nutritional value as compared to brightly colored foods. When selecting breads, make sure the first ingredient listed says whole grain.

🍰 Eat breakfast every single day within one hour of waking up, and make sure it's balanced. You'll want to include some protein, dairy and carbs to help jumpstart your metabolism. It will also keep you from feeling hungry all morning, which will cause you to overeat at lunch.

🍰 A slip-up doesn't mean you should go crazy the rest of the day. Stop, drink a glass of water, forgive yourself and get right back on track for the next meal.

🍰 Don't have more than one big meal in each day. If you plan on having a bigger meal that day, cut back on the other two.

🍰 Eating too little can backfire. Never start a plan that encourages you to eat less than 1300-2000 calories per day for women (depending on your height and weight) and 2000-2600 per day for men without checking with your doctor or nutritionist first. Not eating enough will make your body start clinging to calories rather than burning them.

🍰 Plan around big days. If there is a big party, celebration, or even date coming up, be smart the rest of your day. This doesn't mean to eat less, it means to eat smart. Try an egg-white omelet with veggies for breakfast, and maybe steamed fish and veggies for lunch. This will leave a good amount of calories left to splurge with at your get-together. You could even get an extra workout in to help you out a bit, too.

Part 2: Home

Chances are, you spend most of your eating time at home, and, if you keep not-so-healthy choices in your home, it will make your weight loss efforts a little more difficult.

The best thing you can do is to give your home a weight loss makeover. We see it on the weight loss TV shows all the time! They come in, throw out all the "crap," and fill it up with good healthy choices.

Think about it. If you don't have cookies, processed foods, and other unhealthy foods in your home, it will be much more difficult to eat those things. On the flip side, if you don't have fruits and vegetables in your home, it will be much more difficult to eat those as well.

If you are craving a piece of chocolate, that's totally fine. But having it in your house will make it way too easy to indulge. Letting yourself sit on it for a while will usually make the craving go away. If not, you can always make the trip out to go get it. At least now you know that you were _really_ craving it, and it wasn't a spur of the moment decision just because you were looking at it.

🍰 Keep measuring cups and healthy cooking appliances on the counter, and easy to get to.

🍰 If you have an empty kitchen, (maybe you travel a lot, or you eat out every day, or you just don't know how to cook or like to cook) find a few things that you can keep around for emergencies. Weight loss can happen in restaurants, but it is important that you have healthy options at home for when you're starving and not in the mood to go out. You don't want to get desperate and reach for an old box of mac and cheese just because it's the only thing you can find.

🍰 Leave serving dishes of less-healthy items on the stove rather than placing them family-style on the kitchen table. It's so much easier to avoid sneaking extra bites that way.

🍰 This strategy is opposite for healthy items. Place big dishes of healthy veggies on the table to encourage you and your family to fill up on those foods rather then getting seconds of mashed potatoes.

In the Fridge

It is said that the average person opens the refrigerator and/or freezer door 22 times per day. That is not a little bit! And if your fridge is full of temptations, it may be difficult to work with. Try some of these tips and tricks to keep your fridge a safe zone.

🍰 Throw out everything that is expired.

🍰 Take all of your fruits and veggies out of the drawers!! Everything that is healthy that you want to be attracted to should be front-and-center in your fridge.

🍰 Cut and prep everything! The day you spend shopping, give yourself an extra hour or so to come home and prep your fruits and veggies for the week. Most likely, if you have a giant stalk of celery uncleaned, in the produce bag, hiding in the drawer, then you will *never* eat it! Then, it goes bad, you toss it out, and get upset that you "wasted food," and then never buy celery again.

🍰 Have a giant container (or zip-lock bag if you are interested in saving yourself the dishes) with prepped veggies for your steamer. Baby carrots, zucchini, squash, broccoli and cauliflower are great basics.

🍰 Use small containers for diced up veggies for your cooking. Onions, tomatoes, mushrooms, jalapeños, zucchini, squash, celery, shaved corn off the cob, green onions, and broccoli. These are great for several things including salads, quick soups, veggie omelets, and other recipes.

🍰 To keep your fruits and veggies fresh, look for a product called Bluapple®. The Bluapple® is designed to provide effective ethylene gas absorption for three months in a typical home refrigerator, produce bin or storage container. Search for it on the web!

🍰 Label all of the food in your fridge with a number according to your weight loss plan. This could be in calories, points, grade, or net carbs. Just grab a black sharpie and mark your container. This makes scanning and making decisions easier while on your plan.

🍰 If you live with other people who aren't being as healthy as you are, keep their foods in the drawers, or in the back of the fridge. Or, even better, they get to use the spare fridge in the garage.

🍰 Your healthy foods should be in clear containers. Other tempting foods for family members and roommates should be in opaque containers or wrapped in foil.

🍰 When possible, buy items that are already pre-portioned for you, like yogurt.

🍰 Put left overs in single-serving containers, it will keep your portions in check the next day when you're hungry and the left-over lasagna is calling your name.

In the Pantry

Much like your fridge, you'll want an organized and labeled pantry or cupboards.

🍰 Have a "his and hers," or "kids and adult," separate cupboards so you don't have to stare at their not-so-healthy foods every time you open the door.

🍰 Again, label everything with a number according to your weight loss plan. This could done be in calories, points, grade, or net carbs. This makes scanning and making decisions easier while on your plan.

🍰 Label with YOUR portion size. For instance, if when you pour yourself a bowl of cereal, chances are you aren't pouring the serving size of half a cup. It's probably more like one to two cups. Measure out what your portion size is and use that amount to figure out your calories, points, or other number to label your food with.

🍰 Portion out foods that aren't already pre-portioned. Take your bag of baked chips or crackers, count out how many per portion, put them in individual zip-lock bags, and put the mini bags back into the big bag. Now, when you reach in, you will grab the smaller portioned bag and not over indulge, and your snack will stay fresh longer.

🍰 Also mark foods that you don't plan on eating. A quick story on how this helped me: I was living with a friend while losing my weight and she liked to have treats like Oreos® in the house. The serving size for Oreos® on the back of the box was two cookies… but really, who stops at two Oreos®?! I figured that I would probably eat 10 cookies if I decided to give in to the temptation. So, I put the count for 10 cookies on the front of the box, and while scanning the pantry for something to eat, it made it so much easier to skip the high number on the Oreos® and grab one of my snacks that displayed such a friendlier number marked on the package.

🍰 Do your best to get rid of foods (especially trigger foods) that don't need to be in the house. It's too easy to let yourself indulge when you really don't want to when you have these types of foods in the house.

🍰 If you're buying other snacks for your kids or others in the household, do your best to buy things that you aren't going to be tempted by. Who knows? Maybe you'll help your spouse or kids get healthier, too!

Measuring And Portioning

One of the biggest mistakes people make when journaling their food is that they guesstimate portion sizes rather than measure foods out. This will only hurt you in the end.

Test yourself right now. Pull out the bowl you like to eat cereal in. Pour yourself a bowl (the size you normally would for breakfast) and guess how many cups or ounces it is. Then pour that bowl into a large measuring cup to test your answer. Then compare that pour with the portion size listed on the box. Chances are, unless you are a professional cook, you'll be way off.

🍰 A food scale is extremely helpful. This will help you measure out very accurate portion sizes in grams and ounces. You are even able to set it at zero after placing an empty bowl or plate on it before adding the food, so as not to count the weight of the bowl in your measurement. Very spiffy!

🍰 Have several sets of measuring tools handy. Don't let yourself use the excuse that all of your measuring cups and spoons are dirty or in the dishwasher.

🍰 Find a bowl that has lines or marks inside that you can use as a guide when pouring a bowl of cereal, soup, etc.

🍰 The same goes with wine glasses. There are sets of beautiful glasses with decorative lines around the glass that you can use to measure your wine pours.

🍰 Buy foods that are already portioned when possible.

TV Munching

I get it… You get home from a long day at work, and you just want to crash out on the couch and munch on some junk. Here are some suggestions to enjoy your couch time without overdoing it.

First of all decide if you would rather make the couch a "no food zone" altogether, or if you would rather find ways to make it a healthier environment.

Then figure out <u>why</u> you are tempted to eat in front of the TV or computer. Are you truly hungry? Or are you bored? Or do you just need something to distract your hands?

🍰 Portion Control is huge! Instead of sitting down with a giant bag of chips, figure out how many you can "afford" (which should already be labeled on your bag) and count them out into a bowl or plate. It's so much easier to stop when you're not staring at the open bag.

46

🍰 Find snacks that are lower in calories or fit your specific plan. Fruits and veggies are always good choices. Add some hummus, tzatziki or light ranch made with greek yogurt. That's right, greek yogurt ranch. It's soooo yummy!! Find it in the refrigerated produce section near the bags of salad.

🍰 Chew gum, or brush your teeth before sitting down to watch TV. Something about that minty flavor in your mouth makes it so much easier to not want to eat.

🍰 Find a low calorie or sugar free hard candy to suck on during your show.

🍰 Drink a lot of water.

🍰 Find foods that take a longer time to eat. Peeling an orange keeps your hands busy, or even playing with a light string cheese.

🍰 Find something else to do with your hands rather than shove food in your face. Playing on your laptop or tablet, painting your nails, drawing or doodling, even doing crunches or other mellow exercises in front of the TV.

🍰 You may even want to set a specific time for your kitchen to be "closed for business." No more food is served after "closing time."

🍰 If you know you're going to want something at the end of the day, plan for it that morning, and set aside a specific amount of calories for your TV munching.

🍰 Do your best to fast forward or avoid those commercials. Those images of food will stimulate your hunger, and make it harder to steer clear of temptation.

Snacks

Snacks are important for healthy weight loss. They keep you from overindulging during your meals. The trick is to find snacks that are low in calories yet filling enough to hold you over till your next meal.

Fruits and veggies are a given. You'll want to find ways to keep them interesting. Steam veggies, make salads, or indulge in a delicious veggie soup.

Pair fruits or veggies with some sort of dairy or protein. Fat free and low fat cheese snacks are great. Low calorie string cheese, or Babybel® cheese wedges are fantastic to pair with a sliced apple.

Berries with Light Cool Whip® is a delicious sweet snack. Or drizzle a little honey over plain yogurt to dip your berries in.

🍰 Top light yogurt with your favorite fresh berries. Be cautious with granola. Granola is pretty high in calories, especially if it is sweetened (most are.)

🍰 Put together your own 100-calorie snack bags. There are recipes and ideas all over the internet.

🍰 Fresh almond butter is great, but make sure you are measuring it out and not just spreading a bunch on your bread or celery, as the calories and fat add up easily.

🍰 Veggie chips aren't always a good substitute to potato chips. They are usually made with sweet potatoes and other starchy veggies, <u>and</u> they're often high in fatty oils. Go for some sort of baked chips, and count them out before you start "going to town."

🍰 Granola bars are an easy on-the-go snack.

🛖 Air-popped popcorn is a fantastic snack, especially if you are in a "munchy" mood.

🛖 Shrimp cocktail is super easy and super healthy.

🛖 Laughing Cow® light cheese wedges stuffed in mini bell peppers then baked or grilled is oh so delicious!

🛖 Laughing Cow® light cheese wedges with your favorite baked or light crackers.

🛖 Steamed edamame. You can find frozen single serving packs in your grocer's freezer aisle.

🛖 A small handful of your favorite healthy nuts make for a great dose of protein as a mid-day snack.

Sweets

It's funny how for some people, as soon as you decide to be healthy, sweet foods start calling your name. The only way to stay sane while losing weight is to allow some flexibility. An easy way to accomplish this is to find substitutes that are easier on your body than your old favorites.

🍰 Freezing fruit is an easy way to get that sweet cold fruity taste. Pop a few grapes, pineapple slices, strawberries, or even a banana on a skewer and throw it in the freezer. You could even drizzle a little chocolate syrup or hazelnut spread on the fruit before freezing it.

🍰 Both Weight Watchers® and Skinny Cow® have amazing options in the ice-cream aisle. You could also choose a frozen yogurt instead.

🍰 Skinny Cow® also has candy bar type snacks. If these aren't hitting the spot, attack one or two "fun size" candies rather than getting a full size candy bar.

🍰 You can also find low-calorie brownies, cakes, and other snacks at the grocery store. They are usually in the bread aisle, but every store is set up differently. The chocolate cakes and brownies are even better if you pop them in the microwave for about 10 seconds.

🍰 Fat-free whipped cream is a great tool for sweets. You can mix that with equal parts of your favorite light yogurt. Top with some berries, chopped almonds and a little extra dab of the fat free whipped cream and you have a great sweet treat.

🍰 Marshmallows aren't too bad. If you're around the campfire, don't feel guilty for having a couple.

🍰 Hard candies are relatively low in calories, and they take a while to suck on, so you don't eat as much. These are great for when you are sitting in front of the TV, on a road trip, or while working on the computer.

🍰 Sugar-free gum can also be used for keeping your mouth busy, just like the hard candies do.

🍰 Portion yourself a small serving of dessert if it's really calling your name. Usually just a bite or two will satisfy your sweet tooth.

🍰 Just say no to high calorie sweets that aren't that good. They're not worth it.

Part 3: Shopping and Cooking

🍰 First of all, never shop on an empty stomach. Everything will look so good, and it will be harder to avoid putting unhealthy foods into your cart.

🍰 Also, try to avoid stores and times of the day that constantly have samples out. Yes, samples have calories too, and they add up!

🍰 Go with a plan. Have a list of the foods you need for the week. Have items for snacks, meals, and recipes written on your list and stick to it.

🍰 If you find it hard to stick to your list, take a specific amount of cash with you, or send the spouse or your kid to do the shopping instead.

🍰 Plan on shopping often, at least once a week so you always have fresh fruits and veggies in the house.

🍰 Shop around the perimeter of the grocery store first. This is where you will find all the fresh foods. The junk is always in the middle.

🍰 Start with the vegetables and fruit. Move around to the dairy products then over to the seafood and meats. When you get to the Deli and Bakery, proceed with caution.

🍰 After you've done the bulk of your shopping on the outside of the store, quickly fill in the blanks with the items in the aisles. The frozen section is a great place to end so your food stays frozen until you get home.

🍰 Eating at home is the easiest way to control what you are consuming. You have 100% power over the ingredients that you are putting into your recipes. Cook smart, and save the indulging for special occasions or "date night" at your favorite restaurant.

🍰 While cooking, use tiny coffee spoons for sampling.

🍰 Have a plate of fruits and/or veggies off to the side to munch on while you're cooking.

🍰 Always have a glass of water handy. Make it a fancy water by drinking it out of a wine or cocktail glass. It's more fun that way!

🍰 Play your favorite music in the background to keep yourself moving and burning calories!

Reading Labels

When scanning the labels, there are a few guidelines you will want to know and understand.

Extra lean: Can be used to describe the fat content of meat, game meat, poultry, and seafood. Less than five grams fat, less than two grams saturated fat, and less than 95 milligrams cholesterol per RACC (Reference Amount Customarily Consumed) and per 100 grams.

Lean: Can be used to describe the fat content of meat, game meat, poultry, and seafood. Less than 10 grams fat, less than 4.5 grams saturated fat, and less than 95 milligrams cholesterol per RACC and per 100 grams.

Fresh: Can be used only on raw food that has never been frozen or heated and has no preservatives.

Low: May be used on foods that can be eaten frequently without exceeding dietary guidelines. Per labeled serving and per RACC, these amounts are defined as:

Low calorie: 40 calories or less.

Low cholesterol: Less than 20 milligrams of cholesterol (cholesterol claims are only allowed when saturated fat is two grams or less.)

Low fat: three grams or less of fat.

Low saturated fat: one gram or less of saturated fat and 15 percent or less of calories from saturated fat.

Low sodium: Less than 140 milligrams of sodium.

🍰 Make sure you take a look at the serving size. Many items that look like a single serving (Like a bottle of juice) are really two to three servings, so you'll want to double or triple what the label is telling you to get an accurate count of what you will be consuming.

🍰 Beware of tricky wording. Just because something is low in fat doesn't mean it's low in calories. Often times there will be added sugars or carbs that will bump the calories right back up. And visa versa. When something says it's low in carbs, there may be an excess amount of fat.

🍰 You'll also want to keep an eye open for an abundant amount of sodium. Many weight loss plans don't talk about the sodium in foods very often, but it's not something you want too much of either.

Shopping Substitutions

There are so many things you can substitute at the grocery store. Each little choice can save you a huge amount of calories in your everyday choices.

🍰 Find light versions of all of your dairy products. Skim milk, fat-free or sugar-free creamer, low-fat or fat free cheeses- including cream cheese, cottage cheese, grated cheese, sliced cheese and string cheese. Fat free yogurt or greek yogurt, low-fat or fat-free ranch and other dressings are also substitutes to look for. BTW- Kraft fat-free grated mild cheddar is an amazing fat-free substitute for cheese. It tastes great and even melts just as well as regular cheeses. Also, look for ranch and other dressings made with greek yogurt in the produce section by the bags of lettuce.

🍰 Look for whole-wheat choices instead of white breads, tortillas and pasta. Even better if whole wheat is the first thing listed in the ingredients.

🍰 Labels that show that something high in fiber CAN be a good thing, but if you are a calorie counter, realize that if something is higher in fiber, it is also quite a bit higher in carbs, and it doesn't always balance out to be lighter on the count.

🍰 English muffins are also a great substitute for bread.

🍰 When looking for canned foods, if you have the option to pick ones that are canned in water rather than juices or oils- those will be the lighter choices.

🍰 Look for labels that say lean or extra lean when picking out meats.

🍰 White meats are generally lighter than dark meats are.

🍰 Corn tortillas are usually healthier than flour tortillas, but Mission does have a great whole-wheat tortilla. Just pick the smaller taco-sized tortillas rather than the burrito-sized tortillas.

🍰 Attack the light ice creams for a great low calorie treat. Skinny Cow® and Weight Watchers® both have *amazing* treats.

🍰 100-calorie packs can be smart, but they're not always the healthiest foods. Moderation is key. You don't want to be eating those every day... but once in a while, we all need a taste of sweet.

Cooking Substitutions

So many substitutions can be made while cooking to make your everyday favorite recipes lower in calories and/or fat. Try some of these substitutions with your favorite recipes.

If the recipe calls for:	Then try substituting with:
Bacon	Canadian bacon, turkey bacon, lean prosciutto
Breadcrumbs	Rolled Oats
Butter, margarine or oil to prevent sticking to a pan	Cooking spray, fat free chicken broth, high quality non-stick skillet with splashes of water

If the recipe calls for:	Then try substituting with:
Butter, margarine, shortening or oil in Baked goods	Applesauce for half of the called-for "butter" type ingredient (may need to reduce liquids in recipe), mashed bananas, yogurt, or a light butter substitute
Chicken	Boneless, skinless chicken breast, remove all the excess fat
Cream	Fat-free half-and-half
Cream for soups	Puree steamed cauliflower and/or zucchini, or evaporated milk

If the recipe calls for:	Then try substituting with:
Eggs	Egg substitute or egg whites
Frosting	Marshmallow fluff
Ground beef	Extra-lean ground beef, ground chicken, or ground turkey or use vegetables, beans or whole grains to substitute part on the meat
Mashed potatoes	Mashed cauliflower (do half and half if you prefer)
Sausage	Turkey or chicken sausage
Spaghetti or pasta	Spaghetti squash, or whole wheat pasta

If the recipe calls for:	Then try substituting with:
Sugar	Sugar substitute (Stevia), applesauce, or extra vanilla extract
Sour cream, cream cheese	Non-fat plain greek yogurt. Drain the yogurt overnight to make it thicker for recipes calling for cream cheese. (Yogurt cheese) Just place a paper towel over a colander with a bowl underneath for the drippings. Keep in the fridge
Tuna packed in oil	Tuna packed in water
Vegetable oil	Olive / flaxseed oil, other healthy oils

Veggie Soup

This simple but yummy soup is an easy way to incorporate more vegetables into your day. It's so easy to make in giant batches, and you can even freeze part of it in individual containers for later weeks.

- 1 spray cooking spray

- ½ cup carrots, sliced

- 1 jalapeño, seeded, diced

- ½ cup onions, chopped

- 1 clove garlic, minced

- 2 16 oz. cans of fat free chicken, beef or vegetable broth

- 1 can water

- 1 Tbsp. tomato paste

- ½ tsp. dried basil

- ½ tsp. dried oregano

- ¼ tsp. cayenne pepper

- ¼ tsp. chili powder

- ½ cup broccoli florets

- 1 ear of corn,

- 1 small potato, diced

- ¼ cup zucchini, diced

- ¼ cup squash, diced

- ¼ cup mushrooms, sliced

- ¼ cup tomatoes, diced

- ¼ cup green onions, diced

Spray a skillet with cooking spray; heat. Sauté carrots until they start to get soft – about 4 minutes. Add the minced garlic, jalapeños, and onions. Sauté until onions start to get translucent.

Transfer sautéed vegetables into a giant pot. Add the chicken broth, water, tomato paste and other seasonings. Also add the corn, broccoli, and potatoes.

Bring to a boil, then reduce heat; simmer, covered, about 15 minutes.

Stir in zucchini, squash, mushrooms, tomatoes, and green onions; cook 3-5 minutes more.

Other options:

🍰 Leave out the jalapeños, cayenne pepper, and chili powder if you don't prefer spicy.

🍰 Grill bell peppers with the onions, garlic, and jalapeños.

🍰 Add shredded chopped cabbage and chopped spinach with the corn, broccoli and potatoes.

🍰 Grill and season one chicken breast, dice, and add with the corn, broccoli and potatoes.

🍰 Find other vegetables like Brussels sprouts, asparagus, or snap peas to experiment with.

🍰 Add other seasonings like salt, pepper, even thyme and rosemary for a different flavor.

Part 4: Restaurants

If restaurants make you nervous, you are not alone! With the many people I've coached, restaurants seem to be that one place where they feel out of control on what goes on their plate, and ultimately in their body.

When you're cooking at home, you get to decide what ingredients go into your recipes, what substitutes you want to make, and how much sauce you pour over your meal.

In a restaurant, it's a little different, but it doesn't have to be that intimidating. It just takes a different mindset and a different approach when ordering.

The truth is that you can make healthy decisions in almost <u>every</u> environment where choices are available.

I lost the majority of my weight in restaurants. I was a single bartender, a not-so-amazing cook, and extremely social. I spend a lot of time in restaurants and bars, and I learned how to make them work for me rather than against me. You can, too!

The Basics of Dining Healthy

These are some easy, simple choices you can make while dining out.

🍰 Plan your other meals around the meal you are eating at a restaurant. If you ate out for lunch, plan on making a light meal for dinner. If you know that you have big plans for that night, eat smarter during breakfast and lunch.

🍰 Share a plate with a friend. Most restaurants give portions that are way too big for one person. They also have the portions backwards. While the USDA suggests that half of your plate should be filled with fruits and vegetables, and less than a quarter of the plate should be the protein, you rarely see these kinds of servings in restaurants. Try ordering a plate to share, as well as an extra side of steamed veggies or a garden salad to get the vegetable serving your body really needs.

🍰 If you can't share a plate with a friend, ask the server to bring you a box right at the beginning of the meal so you can put half of it away for later before you start eating. It's so much easier to stop when you're not staring at the food on your plate.

🍰 If you decided to splurge a bit, and you know that taking half home isn't a good idea either, put half of it on a side plate and ruin it with a heaping pile of salt or other table condiment so you won't be tempted to eat it.

🍰 You could even just ask the server to take it away before you start on your half. Remember, you're still wasting food if you eat more than your body requires to function. You're just wasting it in your body, and it does a lot more harm there than it does in the trash.

🍰 Wear tight clothes or a tight belt. The feeling of restriction will send "full" signals to your brain, and keep you from overdoing it.

🍰 Try to plan ahead what you will be eating before you show up at a restaurant. Know how many calories you plan on spending, as well as the kinds of choices you plan on making. You can help yourself with this by looking up the menu online before you go.

🍰 Order a low calorie salad, side of fruit, or bowl of veggie soup that you can fill up on before your meal comes. Be sure to down a glass of water as well.

🍰 Eat slowly. Give your stomach time to tell your brain when it's full.

🍰 Eat with chopsticks when you can. It will help you eat slower, and it's fun!

🍰 Look for à la carte items and/or appetizers. They are usually smaller portions, and you can mix and match them to get a good amount of veggies in.

🍰 Shrimp cocktail is a fantastic appetizer. It takes time to peel and eat, and no one will ever know you're consciously eating healthy.

Scan the Menu

There are a few things to look out for when you scan a menu at any restaurant.

🍰 Watch out for scary words like fried, cheesy, rich, crispy, au gratin, pan fried, rich, and creamy.

🍰 Look for words like fresh, steamed, broiled, lean, low fat, whole wheat and whole grain.

🍰 White meats are generally lower in calories than dark meats. Chicken, turkey, and white fish can be great choices if they are prepared the right way.

🍰 If you're in the mood for steak, filet mignon usually has the least amount of fat on the cut. Make sure you ask them not to brush it with butter.

🍰 Look at the side(s) that come with your meal. Look for healthier options like fresh fruit, steamed veggies, or a green salad to substitute.

🍰 At a buffet, do a round before filling your plate. Decide what looks the best before filling your plate with those so-so items that you really don't want. Start with a healthy green salad, and then when you fill your dinner plate make sure half of your plate is filled with fruits and vegetables.

🍰 Be the first of your friends to order so you're not tempted by their choices, and so you're more inclined to make the requests you want. Often, some of your friends will follow suit to be healthy with you, so you can be an inspiration!

🍰 Pass on the bread. Unless it's your favorite part of the meal. If you do decide you're in the mood for bread, decide what you choose to give up in it's place. This may be the cheese on your entrée, or the glass of wine you've been thinking about. It's all about balance.

Questions to Ask Your Server

I've worked in restaurants for almost 15 years of my life, and I promise you, any good server is happy to help you find something on the menu that you would enjoy. Most restaurants do a great job training their employees about the details of the menu. Some restaurants even train their servers to recite the recipes for each sauce the kitchen serves. Don't be afraid or embarrassed to ask questions!

🍰 Ask the hostess for the nutritional menu. You'd be surprised at how many restaurants offer these now upon request. You can always look it up online before you go as well. It really helps to make smart choices when you're looking right at the calorie count.

🍰 Ask your server to have the chef hold any extra butter. They often spread butter on food to make it look fresh, to make it glisten, or to add flavor. This happens most often on veggies, fish and steaks.

🍰 Order any sauces or dressings on the side. This way you control how much goes on your food. Those little dressing containers are usually two fluid ounces, and the larger ones are usually four fluid ounces. The dressing boats are even more.

🍰 Modify your dish by removing any toppings, cheeses or sauces that may be higher in calories. Make sure you still enjoy the dish. If cheese is important to you, leave it. Just find something else that you don't want as much to remove instead. You could even ask for easy cheese or cheese on the side. Add other things like salsa to increase the flavor.

🍰 Ask your server if there are healthier options available. Especially with dressings and sauces.

◤ Ask your server the portion size of meats and other items to find out how to journal your selection.

◤ Substitute a starchy side dish for extra veggies, a garden salad, or fruit.

◤ Ask your server to keep your water glass full throughout the meal, and drink it!

The Myth On Salads

I'm sure you have "a friend" (I *promise* I'm not talking about you) who at some point in their life, maybe even now, think that if they order any salad off of the menu they are eating healthy, or taking in less calories than if they ordered pizza or a burger. In some cases this is true, but most salads are <u>full</u> of hidden (and sometimes obvious) calories that may do more damage than good.

I've seen salads at fast food restaurants that ended up being more calories than a cheeseburger and fries. Salads can be a great weight loss tool if used correctly, just proceed with caution using these tips.

🍰 Watch out for cheeses, croutons, wonton strips, tortilla strips, nuts, seeds, avocado, meats, bacon, eggs, beans, and especially dressings. Now, I'm not saying that all of those toppings are bad, I'm just saying that they will all add calories to your salad that you may not be aware of.

82

🍰 Some cheeses are fewer calories than others. Most are around 100-120 calories per ounce, but feta cheese, soft goat cheese, and part-skim mozzarella (which is the most widely used mozzarella) are around 75 calories per ounce. You may prefer to select a stronger cheese like parmesan of which you will be able to use less of.

🍰 Do your best to find a light dressing. Some plans love olive oil, and vinaigrettes; others aren't so keen on them. Olive oil is a healthy oil, but it is still high in calories. It is a smarter choice than a creamy dressing like ranch or blue cheese, but you will still want to use it sparingly. Most creamy and vinaigrette dressings are around 300 calories for a small two ounce side.

🍰 There is a big difference between vinegar and vinaigrette. Balsamic and red wine vinegar are extremely low in calories, but their vinaigrette siblings have quite a bit of oil in them, which also means more calories.

🍰 Dressings should always come on the side so you can control how much goes into your salad.

🍰 When ordering a large dinner size salad, ask them to put the dressing in a small ramekin or two ounce container, rather than the big four ounce ramekin or container. It's much easier to measure the amount of dressing you end up using.

🍰 If there isn't a low calorie dressing on the menu, ask for a side of ranch as well as a side of salsa or buffalo sauce. When you mix the two together, you end up with a delicious spicy dressing. It's only half the calories, and the flavor is stronger so you can use less. Buffalo or wing sauce is usually made of peppers, unless it's a sweetened wing sauce. Many restaurants use the standard Frank's® RedHot® Cayenne Pepper Sauce which is only 5 calories per serving.

🍰 Try dipping your fork into the dressing first before stabbing the greens. It gives you that flavor but avoids the unnecessary calories when you dip your greens into the dressing.

🍰 Foods like eggs, beans, nuts, seeds, and avocado can be good choices depending on your plan. They are full of fiber and very filling, and have benefits for your body.

🍰 Whatever you do, pass on the cobb salad. It is topped with piles of bacon, cheese and eggs, and very minimal vegetables.

🍰 When looking up nutritional values for the salads at restaurants, they almost always show the calorie count without the dressing included. Make sure you find the calories for the dressing to find the grand total.

🍰 Salads are a great weight loss tool *if* you do them the right way. Stick with veggies and lean proteins and you are good to go.

85

American Restaurants and Steakhouses

Have you ever noticed how most "American" restaurants have a little bit of everything on the menu? You will often see pasta, tacos, and rice bowls, as well as burgers, steaks, fish and chicken wings. There may be quite a few choices, but almost always a handful of good choices.

🍰 Sometimes appetizers are a good idea, depending on what's offered. It's usually smaller portions, so if you can steer clear of all the fried stuff, they are often times great choices. Ceviche, edamame, lettuce cups, mussels, clams, shrimp cocktail, veggie tray, ahi sashimi… the list goes on.

🍰 Pair an appetizer with a small salad, cup of veggie soup, or side of steamed veggies.

🍰 If you are craving a dip like hummus, or tzatziki, but you want to pass on the bread that is served with it, ask for a side of sliced cucumbers or tomatoes to dip with instead of the bread.

🍰 If you are ordering a melt or panini, ask if they butter the bread before they grill it. Find out if there is a way to avoid that.

🍰 Scan the menu for other healthy options, like street tacos, turkey sandwiches (hold the mayo), grilled chicken or fish, even lean steaks like filet mignon. Always ask for sauces on the side, and select smart sides.

🍰 Watch out for sandwiches with a ton of meats and cheeses piled on. Three to four ounces of meat is plenty. One ounce of deli meat or sliced cheese is about the same size of a CD. Imagine three to four of those on your sandwich, with one slice of cheese, and that is plenty. Still watch out for creamy dressings. Spread avocado on the bread for moisture, and use mustard instead of mayo.

🍰 Veggie burgers aren't necessarily lighter options. They usually bulk them up with rice or soy (most of which can lead to estrogen dominance and cause belly-fat). Sometimes, if you are counting calories, a simple grilled chicken breast is the best substitution for a burger.

🍰 If you're craving a burger, go after the kid-sized burger instead of the half-pound patty on the adult menu. Ketchup and mustard are extremely low in calories, so use those condiments instead of dressing like ranch, mayo or thousand island. Pass on the fries, and go for a baked potato or salad instead.

🍰 Top your potato with steamed vegetables with salsa or chili instead of sour cream, butter, bacon, cheese or ranch.

🍰 Nice steakhouses are a great place to indulge in a fantastic piece of fish. They usually offer a nice big plump cut, and if you ask, they will prepare it extremely healthy for you.

Mexican

OLÉ! Time for a little flavor from south of the border. While many people who are counting calories get the jitters when facing the menu of cheese drenched fried foods, there are options that are super minimal and extremely healthy!

🍰 Street tacos are your new best friend. A simple taco with a corn tortilla, a few ounces of meat, topped with salsa and other veggies is always a great choice! Watch out for cream sauces and cheeses. Of course, a little sprinkle isn't awful, but not always necessary.

🍰 Skip the combo plates and check out the à la carte menu. Unless you love rice and beans and it's worth the extra 200+ calories each, per cup, you don't really need them on your plate. If you do order a combination, find out if they offer steamed veggies or a garden salad as a substitute for rice.

🍰 Whole black beans (210 calories per cup) are much healthier than refried beans (370 calories per cup). Ask them not to sprinkle the cheese on top for a more guilt-free side item.

🍰 Fajitas can be a good choice, but ask them if it is possible to use little- to no oil. Some restaurants like their fajitas veggies swimming in oil, and that builds up the unnecessary calories. You may even want to get extra pico de gallo and guacamole instead of cheese and sour cream.

🍰 Corn tortillas are fewer calories than flour tortillas. Plus, it's hard to find wheat tortillas in restaurants.

🍰 Burrito size tortillas contain a truckload of calories. Burrito bowls are so much smarter, and if you want the tortilla flavor, ask for a taco-sized tortilla on the side.

🍰 If the chips and salsa are too tempting to pass up, count out the amount that you are willing to spend your calories on and put them on your plate. You can even take your few chips and break them up so you end up with a bunch of mini chips! This let's you munch while waiting for your food, take more bites, but eat less chips.

🍰 If they are giving out tri-colored chips, call dibs on all of the "red" chips and stick to your guns! You'll eat fewer than if you were just grabbing any colored chips.

🍰 Salsas and hot sauces are just vegetables and are "free" on many weight loss plans, so pile them on for flavor.

Italian

Italian food can be intimidating, but with a little knowledge and pre-planning, you'll be able to enjoy a delicious meal.

🍰 Italian restaurants are notorious for serving gigantic portions. A serving of pasta should be no more than one cup, and we both know that the giant bowl of pasta they serve is way more than a cup. Practice portion control, or share a plate.

🍰 Gravitate towards a red sauce over a white sauce. Alfredo and other creamy sauces are quite a bit higher in calories.

🍰 Pick a dish that has a lot of vegetables in with it. They will usually use less pasta to make room for the veggies.

🍰 Ask them not to sprinkle extra cheese on top. You may even want to ask them to hold any extra cheese they use while cooking. Often times they will add the extra cheese while putting together the pasta, sauce, veggies and protein.

🍰 Search for a pasta free dish. Many restaurants serve a simple plate that comes with a side of pasta or potatoes. Substitute the starch for extra steamed vegetables instead.

🍰 Find out if they offer whole wheat pasta as a slightly healthier option.

🍰 Order a "skinny pizza" Ask them to make the crust ultra paper thin and go easy on the cheese, then top with all of your favorite veggies. One slice is usually less than 200 calories!

🍰 Before starting, decide which parts of the meal are the most important to you. Is it the bread? The cocktails? An appetizer? Dessert? Pick where you decide to splurge, and say no to the rest. If a glass of wine is more important to you than a breadstick, go for that, and be content with your choice.

Sushi

We all know that sushi can be extremely healthy for you, if done right. The trick is to go for the whole foods and passing on the white rice, deep-fried rolls and items covered in spicy mayo.

🍰 Edamame! It's a high calorie vegetable, but still extremely healthy. Watch out for sauces and marinades that many restaurants will offer like "garlic edamame" that may be dripping in oil.

🍰 If you still haven't heard of rice-free cucumber rolls, these will change your life! MOST sushi restaurants offer a sushi roll that has no rice and is wrapped in cucumber. They are *delicious*, and oh so healthy.

🍰 Steer clear of tempura anything. This is just a fancy word for deep-fried.

🍰 Always ask for low-sodium soy sauce.

🍰 Miso soup is a great low calorie starter.

🍰 Instead of nigiri, just order sashimi. It's the same thing, usually a larger slice, and without the rice. Remember that rice acts like a sponge with the soy sauce, and even with low-sodium soy, rice will suck it up and all that extra salt will make your body retain water.

🍰 Skip the sake, and stick with your favorite light beer, wine or cocktail. A six ounce serving of sake has about 230 calories. A six-ounce glass of wine has about 150 calories. The choice seems simple.

Fast Food

We all know that fast food isn't the healthiest choice available, but there are some choices that are better than others.

🍰 Change what you call fast foods. Start looking at Subway®, Flame Broiler, Rubio's®, and other options that are still fast, but don't include a drive-thru. They usually use fresh ingredients that aren't overly processed, and often have better side choices including more vegetables.

🍰 Go for a six-inch instead of that footling. You and I both know you don't *really* need all of that food. Remember, you're goal is to stop eating when you hit a six, not a nine or ten.

🍰 Go for the fat-free condiments like mustard instead of mayo.

🍰 At a joint that has chicken and rice bowls, ask them to go easy on the rice, and throw in the extra vegetables. Go easy on the teriyaki sauce as well.

◣ Opt out of the combo meal with fries. If they offer a salad, fruit, or veggie side as a choice, go that route.

◣ Pick a grilled chicken sandwich over a fried chicken sandwich or a cheeseburger. Lighten it up even more by asking them to hold the mayo and cheese. Also, don't order your chicken "spicy," that's just a cue for them to fry it with spicy seasonings.

◣ Kids meals will be smaller and easier on the calories than adult meals. A kid's cheeseburger is only 275-325 calories, where a quarter pound burger with cheese is 520-750 calories.

◣ Be careful with salads. They can be deceitful. Watch out for croutons, cheeses, fatty meats, crispy strips, and other add-ons. Be especially cautious of dressings. Often a single side of dressing can be the same amount of calories as two slices of pizza!

🍰 When at a fast food taco place, go for tacos over burritos. Those large flour tortillas can be curiously high in calories. Ask them to hold the creamy sauces, sour cream and cheese, then ask them to add pico de gallo or other salsa to bump up the flavor. (Some may call it "fresco style".)

🍰 Wrap a sandwich in lettuce instead of the bread or bun. Or, you could just get rid of half of the bun and eat it open faced. Maybe you even would prefer to tear off and toss some of the bread as you go.

🍰 Skip the fast food shakes, and go for the yogurt parfait instead, or wait till you can get your hands on some frozen yogurt or one of your light options at home.

🍰 If you are at a fried chicken chain, go for a BBQ chicken sandwich, or peel off the breading and skin off of the fried chicken. Obviously you'll want to pair that with veggies. Hold the butter.

Fast Food Comparisons

Most big fast food joints have nutritional menus on their pages that are interactive, so you can add and subtract the toppings to see how you can change the calorie count of your favorite choices.

🍰 McDonald's®

Premium Grilled Chicken Classic Sandwich: 350 calories. Cut the mayo and save an extra 50 calories.

Fruit 'n Yogurt Parfait: 150 calories.

Kid's hamburger: 250 calories.

Premium Bacon Ranch Salad with Grilled Chicken (no dressing): 230 calories. Add half of the ranch packet for 80 calories, or the low fat balsamic, or low fat Italian for 40 calories.

Big Mac: 550 calories.

Quarter Pounder with Cheese: 520 calories.

Premium Crispy Chicken Club Sandwich: 670 calories.

French fries; kids: 100 calories, small: 230 calories, large: 500 calories

🍰 Burger King®

Tendergrill® Chicken Sandwich: 470 calories. Save 90 calories by holding the mayo.

Kid's hamburger: 240 calories

Whopper: 630 calories. Add 50 calories for cheese.

Tendercrisp® Chicken Sandwich: 750 calories.

French fries; Value: 240 calories, small: 340 calories, large: 500 calories.

Chocolate Hand Spun shake: 760 calories.

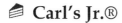 Carl's Jr.®

Charbroiled BBQ Chicken Sandwich™: 390 calories.

Turkey Burger: 490 calories. Hold the mayo to save 110 calories.

Famous Star® with cheese: 670 calories.

Original Six Dollar Burger™: 890 calories.

Bacon Swiss Crispy Hand-breaded Chicken Tender Sandwich™: 570 calories.

French fries; small: 300 calories, large: 460 calories.

Chocolate Hand-Scooped Ice Cream Shake™: 690 calories.

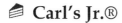 Jack In The Box®

Chicken Fajita Pita: 326 calories.

Jr. Jack™: 324 calories.

Grilled Chicken Salad without dressing or croutons: 245 calories. Add croutons: 50 calories, Bacon Ranch Dressing: 220 calories, Lite Ranch Dressing: 130 calories, Low-Fat Balsamic Vinaigrette: 25 calories.

Jumbo Jack® with Cheese- 572 calories.

Homestyle Ranch Chicken Club- 726 calories.

Two Tacos: 386 calories.

French fries; Value: 225 calories, small: 333 calories, large: 557 calories.

Chocolate Ice Cream Shake; Regular 16 oz.: 798 calories, large 24 oz.: 1147 calories.

🍰 Taco Bell®

Fresco Soft Taco: 160 calories. Chicken: 140 calories.

Fresco Burrito Supreme® Chicken: 340 calories, Steak: 350 calories.

Burrito Supreme: 420 calories.

Grilled Stuft Burrito: 880 calories.

Nachos BellGrande®: 780 calories.

🍰 Del Taco®

Grilled Chicken Soft Taco: 220 calories. Hold the cheese and sauce and add pico de gallo for less calories.

Taco Al Carbon; Chicken or Steak: 150 calories.

Regular Taco: 130 calories.

Del Combo Burrito™: 530 calories.

½ lb. Bean & Cheese Burrito: 470 calories.

MACHO Combo Burrito™: 940 calories.

🍰 Kentucky Fried Chicken

KY Grilled Chicken®; (single item) Breast: 220, Drumstick: 90, Thigh: 170, Wing: 80 calories.

Original Recipe®; (single item) Breast: 360, Drumstick: 120, Thigh: 250, Wing: 120 calories.

Extra Crispy™; (single item) Breast:490, Drumstick: 160, Thigh: 370, Wing: 210 calories.

Biscuit: 180 calories.

Mashed Potatoes: 170 calories.

Coleslaw: 120 calories.

Corn on the Cob: 70 calories.

Brunch and Breakfasts

Breakfast is the most important meal of the day. Many even think that it's better to have your biggest meal in the morning, then a medium sized meal for lunch, and easy snacking for dinner.

Eating a good breakfast will get your metabolism working, and will keep you running throughout the day.

🍰 Remember that brunch is usually about the company that you are with. Make sure that they are your focus, not the pile of muffins in the corner of the buffet.

🍰 Did you know that you can order a "skinny bagel" at most bagel shops? Really! Instead of slicing it once down the middle, they slice it twice then throw the middle part away. Some even have this special tool that makes it super easy.

🍰 Choose fruit or low fat cottage cheese as a side instead of breakfast potatoes or hash browns.

🍰 Look for a vegetarian omelet or scramble on the menu. Then, tweak it a bit by asking them to hold the cheese, and trading the regular eggs for egg whites or egg substitute.

🍰 If you're not into egg whites, order your eggs poached instead of fried, scrambled, or part of a six-egg omelet.

🍰 Salsa is just vegetables, so feel free to pile it on!

🍰 Ask them to go easy on the oil or butter. Or, ask if they can just hold the butter or oil all together.

🍰 Ask them to serve your toast dry. Spread avocado on your toast with a little salt and/or pepper to get some of that healthy fat into your breakfast instead of using butter, jelly or cream cheese.

🍰 If you chose something not so healthy, eat the fruit first and down a glass of water so you don't have as much room for the "splurgy" foods.

🍰 Pick between sweet and savory. If you're really craving both, order a single dry (no butter) pancake à la carte and top it with sugar free syrup (yes, most places have it if you ask) or jam. Or just sneak a bite from your friend's plate.

🍰 If you can't get past that sweet treat, go for the kid's meal version. At least you know the portion will be smaller.

🍰 If you are at a brunch, pass on the Mimosas, and go for a Bloody Mary, or just do the champagne solo. You'll save yourself quite a bit of calories for passing on the orange juice, especially if you plan on having more than one.

🍰 If it's a bottomless glass, ask for a fresh glass instead of topping yours off. It will help you keep track of how much you are actually drinking.

🍰 If it's a brunch buffet, do a lap first to see your options. Thin start with a plate of fruits or a green salad (depending on your mood) before you dig into the other choices.

🍰 Look for sugar-free or fat-free single serving size creamer packets to take with you for your coffee. Using those and a sugar substitute can help you keep your coffee calories extremely low.

Part 5: Drinking Your Calories

I know it's unfair, but your drinks have calories too. Whether you're a coffee drinker, juice drinker, or even an alcohol drinker, it's important that you count those calories, as well.

Unless your plan says to specifically cut drinks out of your plan, there is no need to be afraid to enjoy a night out with your friends.

You've found the right place to get everything you need to know about smart drinks. I've worked behind the bar for a total of nine years, and have done my research on low-calorie drinks.

🍰 The biggest thing to watch out for is the craving for foods when you're not actually hungry after a night out on the town drinking alcohol. If you're going to bed in the near future, you'll be fine. Just pass on the late night munchies, and wait for breakfast. You'll also feel better in the morning.

🍰 Alternate drinks with water or tea. Hot tea is a fantastic choice, especially at pricey restaurants (they have the best tea choices!) They take longer to drink, and many places have several choices including some great fruity caffeine-free herbal teas.

Beer

Just because a beer is darker doesn't make it higher in calories. Guinness at 125 calories for a twelve ounce bottle is actually less than good ol' Budweiser at 145 calories. A bottle of Sierra Nevada is 175 calories, and Corona Extra is 148 calories.

🍰 Light beers are less in calories, and the basic light beers are all within a 10-20 calorie difference at about 90-110 calories each.

🍰 There are a couple of "super light" beers out there. To save the most calories on a beer, look for Miller 64 and Bud Select 55. (64 and 55 calories, respectively)

🍰 To add a little flavor to your light beer, try a teeny tiny splash of orange juice! It sounds interesting, I know, but there's nothing like a "beermosa" on a warm summer day. Crisp, refreshing, and delicious!

🍰 Order bottle beers instead of draft beers. A bottle beer is 12 ounces, where a draft beer is 16 ounces. Be extra cautious of the oversize drafts. A bottle of Bud Light® is 110 calories, but a 16 ounce pint is 147 calories. If you plan on having a few throughout the night, the bottles will really help you stay within your numbers.

Wine

🍰 For you wine drinkers, my biggest piece of advice to you is to know how many ounces your bartender is pouring. Some restaurants pour five ounces, others pour six to seven ounces. After a few glasses, those extra ounces are extra calories that may not be accounted for. Just ask your bartender how many ounces their pour is.

🍰 Use small wine glasses or champagne glasses to stay on top of the ounces poured into your glass.

🍰 There isn't a big difference in the calorie count between red wines and white wines. The higher calories are in the wines with a higher alcohol content.

🍰 Try a spritzer. Half wine, and half soda water on ice. Best when served with a squeeze of your favorite citrus fruit. Orange is a favorite.

🍰 Sangrias are full of sugary juices, so those aren't usually the best choice.

🍰 If you're going for champagne, pass on the orange juice, or ask for it on the side so you can add only a small splash.

Cocktails

🍰 Cocktail drinkers get a few more choices! Clear spirits (vodka, silver tequila, silver rum, gin) are going to be better choices than gold or dark spirits.

🍰 Syrupy and sugary liquors (Peach Schnapps, Midori, Grand Marnier®, etc.) are higher in sugars, which make them high in carbs and calories. So watch out for super-sweet mixed drinks.

🍰 Mixers are usually what make a drink high in calories. Juices, sodas, sweet and sour mix, grenadine, sweetened lime juice, and simple syrup (sugar water) are all extremely high in sugars, and therefor calories.

🍰 If you are counting calories, you may also want to ask your bartender how many ounces their pour is. Many bars and restaurants only pour 1.5 ounces, but others have an extremely generous pour of 3 ounces. This can make a big difference in your overall calorie count.

🍰 Soda water or flat water is always safe. Just squeeze your favorite citrus fruit and you have a safe simple cocktail.

🍰 If you are ok using sugar substitutes (check your diet plan, as they have different opinions about this), there are plenty of other options. Diet cola is always available in bars and restaurants. You can mix this with vodka, or rum. (Try a Malibu® Coconut Rum and diet, it's amazing!)

🍰 You could also buy Crystal Light packets and carry them with you in your pockets, car or purse, and use those in your cocktails. Just mix about a third of a packet to your vodka soda and you have instant flavor! If you're not a fan of carbonation, try vodka water. You could do the same with rum and tequila. They have a bunch of flavors, so you can keep changing the flavor of your cocktail. They even have a margarita flavored mix, so you could mix that with a tequila and water and you have an instant sugar-free low calorie margarita!

🍰 Martini's are also something to look out for. They will either have quite a bit of juice, which is high in sugar, or _a lot_ of alcohol. Traditional martinis are pure liquor, so the pour is high, but will vary restaurant to restaurant. Traditional vodka or gin martinis are a good choice since they don't have any mixers. Just be smart, ask your bartender how many ounces the pour is, and always drink responsibly. :)

🍰 Be careful even when ordering "skinny cocktails." Many bartenders don't know how to make a "skinny margarita," especially if they work in a small bar. Most don't even know what a real skinny margarita is! Many bartenders don't understand that the agave syrup, which should come in a skinny margarita, still has calories, so they will be very generous with it. Many will still add sweet n sour and/or salt, which shouldn't be included in a skinny margarita. You may want to just take matters in your own hands and use the margarita flavored Crystal Light, or ask your bartender if they've been trained on building a skinny margarita.

🍰 If the simple vodka soda types of drinks aren't your type and you need a little more flavor, order a vodka soda (or similar) and add a splash of juice or soda. You could try a vodka soda with a splash of cranberry, orange juice, pineapple juice, lemonade, sprite, or even iced tea. Using mostly soda water or water will save you a ton of calories.

Other Drinks

I get that everyone has different opinions on what is healthy and what isn't. Some are ok with sugar substitutes, others aren't. Some programs encourage you to juice, others prefer you to eat a whole piece of fruit and skip the juicing. Some are ok with caffeine, and some aren't. Here are some general things I have found, take what you like, and ignore what you don't like.

🍰 DRINK LOTS OF WATER!!! ALL THE TIME!!!

🍰 Tea is a great option if you get bored of water. Hot and cold teas are fantastic.

🍰 Crystal Light packets are zero calories, and great to use when you're not in the mood for water.

🍰 Sugar-free sodas are generally calorie free.

🍰 If you don't like the taste of diet sodas, then try doing three parts diet cola and 1 part of cola, root beer, or Dr. Pepper®. I bet you would never taste the difference, and it will save you so many calories. You may even be able to pour mostly diet cola with just a splash of your favorite soda (about one inch at the top of your cup.)

🍰 When drinking your calories, use tall skinny glasses instead of pint glasses or short glasses. It's easier for you to determine the portion this way. Try it at home! Take one of each of your water glasses, wine glasses, coffee mugs (different sizes) and fill them with water how you normally would. Guess how many ounces you poured, then test your guesses with a measuring cup. You may be surprised at your guessing skills.

🍰 If you are in the mood for a smoothie, make sure you are using a fat-free yogurt, and watch out for the amount of juices added.

🍰 Black coffee is calorie free; it's the creamer and sugar that pack on the calories. If you are interested in a super low calorie coffee, check out the sugar-free and fat-free creamers in the refrigerated area at the grocery store. They offer them in all kinds of flavors, and I bet you would never taste the difference. Add a little zero calorie sweetener and you are good to go!

🍰 If you're in the mood for a fancy coffee, ask for a fat free latte/cappuccino. If you want to add flavor, ask them what sugar-free syrups they offer.

🍰 Find out if they have a "light" blended coffee drink. Pass on the whipped cream. You'll survive, I promise.

🍰 While fruit juices may seem like a good idea, you may want to be cautious with them. Especially if it is not freshly juiced. Packaged juices usually contain added sugar and other additives.

Part 6: Other Places

Of course you have other environments that you need a plan for. This may be your car, workplace, or even the ballpark.

Take a look at all of the different environments that you spend time in. Where do you tend to overeat and make not so great eating decisions?

Have a plan for each of those places, and stay in control.

At Work

Obviously everyone has different types of work environments, and the flexibility of the food you can keep in your place of work will vary. Try to take some of these ideas and use them to figure out how you can make your own work environment work a little bit more to your advantage.

🍰 Always eat breakfast before work. It will keep you on your A-game, and will help to keep you from over-indulging on your lunch break. It will also help you choose NOT to indulge on the doughnuts your co-worker so lovingly brought in to share.

🍰 Don't be the employee that keeps the candy dish on your desk. If you insist on it, choose candies that you don't care for. But honestly, my guess is that most of the people you work with probably would love to eat healthier themselves, so do *them* a favor and keep the temptation away.

🍰 If the candy is on another desk, find something else to distract you from the goodies calling your name. If you cave, pick a hard candy that you can suck on while you gossip or catch up with your co-workers.

🍰 Keep your own natural sugar substitutes and fat-free or sugar-free creamers at the office to keep your Cup-o-Joe low in calories. You can even buy the single servings of Coffee-Mate® Sugar Free French Vanilla Creamers. These are easy to keep in your drawer so others don't use them uninvited. The powdered creamers are also low in calories.

🍰 Keep a snack stash of granola bars, nuts, and other snacks in your drawer. Also make it a habit to bring fresh fruit or vegetables with you each day for snacking.

In The Car

So, you just got off work, you're starving, but you have dinner plans in 2 hours. What do you do? Most people will pull into a drive-thru for a "snack." While fast food places can have OK choices, it's not always the best idea for a snack. You'll most likely just end up eating two meals worth of calories in the end.

🍰 Keep a box of granola bars in your car. Try to keep them in a center console or a cooler area that's covered in your trunk.

🍰 Chug a bottle of water. You'd be surprised how often that can fill you up.

🍰 Stop at a grocery store and grab a cup of prepared fresh cut fruit, or a take-out bowl of veggie soup.

🍰 Work on making it a habit to always have a snack with you when leaving the house. Maybe you could just grab a couple 100-calorie bags, or an insulated lunch bag with fresh fruit or veggies.

125

Parties And Celebrations

You don't want to be the person who is eating carrots and celery sticks and crying in the corner. I get it. So don't be! Just make sure that you have a plan, and parties will be super simple.

🍰 Bring a dish to share that you are comfortable eating. Whether it's a fruit or veggie platter, or a low calorie recipe that you've wanted to try out. You don't even have to tell people how healthy it is. I'm sure the one you pick out will be so delicious that people won't even care!

🍰 Talk to the host about what will be served. This will help you decide if you want to bring any low calorie condiments with you for the main dish.

🍰 Don't hang around the food table. It's dangerous. 'Nuff said.

🍰 Bring drink options with you. Either your favorite bottle of wine, a six pack of your super duper light beers, or a box of Crystal Light packets to mix with vodka and water. Now you are good to go!

🍰 Do your best to be the last person to fill your plate at serving time. This way you won't be tempted to go back for seconds, cause you will be the only person still eating.

🍰 Be picky. Pass on things that are available anytime anywhere, and pick things that are special for that occasion. Who needs 3 different kinds of potato salad? The same goes for holiday cookie parties. You don't need the chocolate chip cookies, you can get them anytime! But the gingerbread cookies are seasonal.

🍰 Use the smaller plate to build your meal on if they are offered. Smaller plate = less food = a happier you.

🍰 If you are trying not to over-do it with drinks, play the bracelet or rubber band game! Before you leave for the party, decide how many drinks you are allowing yourself to have, and put that many bracelets or rubber bands on your wrist. Each time you start a new drink, move one to the other wrist (or throw it away.) Once you've run out, you know you're done for the night.

🍰 Volunteer to be the designated driver for the night. Being accountable to others makes it easier to be good.

🍰 When it comes to desserts, you could share one with a friend, *or* make yourself choose between dessert and something else like a drink or an appetizer. Tell yourself you can only have one or the other, and stick to your choice.

🍰 Don't take home the leftovers. (Unless they're healthy.) If you're the one hosting the party, send everything out the door with your guests. Especially anything overly tempting.

Sporting Events, Concerts and Fairs

Hot dogs, nachos, pretzels and beer. What to do?!

🍰 Sneak in your own snacks! But only if you dare to be a little rebellious. If security asks about it at the gate, tell them you're on a strict plan. Many will be cool about it.

🍰 Instead of settling for the basic food cart, search for a cart that has fresh fruit, veggies, or even wraps and sandwiches. Most major sports venues have a bunch of healthy options to pick from. Don't settle for the first food court you see.

🍰 Pick the grilled chicken sandwich over the burger or fried chicken strips. Hold the sauces.

🍰 Drink a lot of water!

🍰 Make it a point to do more walking around, and using the stairs as opposed to the escalators. Earn that beer!

🍰 Hot dogs aren't a horrible choice. The dog on a bun (regular size, not those crazy foot long ones) is only around 300 calories. Top it with ketchup and mustard and you are good to go!

🍰 Don't get too distracted by all of the bacon-wrapped fried foods at the fair. You will always find healthier options like corn on the cob, turkey legs and caramel apples.

🍰 Veggie kebabs anyone?

🍰 Look for booths that sell fresh fruit, other vegetables, and chicken and rice bowls. Ask for easy brown rice and extra veggies of course.

🍰 Find a place that offers grilled chicken. Whether it's on a sandwich or with pineapple and rice.

Vacations

The first thing to decide is what you expect or want to have happen while you are away. Do you plan on losing weight while on vacation, or are you ok with maintaining your weight or possibly gaining a pound or two.

Vacationing can be easy if you follow the tips listed in the restaurants section.

If you've been planning a trip to Italy, and you know you will want to eat more pasta than normal, allow yourself some wiggle room.

This doesn't mean that you need to give yourself a free pass to eat unhealthy at every sitting, but allow yourself to enjoy your vacation. That is what life is all about.

🍰 Eat smart breakfasts as often as possible. If you plan on splurging on later meals, do your best to stick to fruits, oatmeal, and veggie omelets at breakfasts.

🍰 Practice portion control as often as you can. Share meals, don't over eat, and choose smart sides with your meals.

🍰 Remember that you will most likely be moving a lot more while on vacation. Most of us walk quite a bit more while sightseeing. This will help out, but don't count on it to override all of the extra calories you are eating.

🍰 If you go on a cruise, vow to never use the elevator the whole time. Use the stairs no matter how tired you are. It will do amazing things for your body in the end.

🍰 While on a road-trip, take healthy snacks, crackers, and fruits and vegetables with you. When eating meals, choose joints that don't have a drive-thru window. They tend to have healthier choices.

Part 7: Fitness

Obviously fitness plays a big roll in weight loss. The fact is that when you are burning calories, you are on the fast track to hit your goals.

🍰 Change your perspective. Stop calling or thinking of yourself as a lazy couch potato, and start calling yourself fit and an athlete. Even if it's tough at first, keep it up and after a while, you'll start to believe yourself.

🍰 Even if you aren't ready to start hard-core fitness routine, you at least want to start moving more than you are now.

🍰 Muscle mass will actually burn more calories while you are doing nothing, which makes building muscle a double bonus.

🍰 Be sure to get in cardio as well as toning and muscle building. A well-rounded workout plan will do wonders to your body.

🍰 Remember, losing weight will help you look sexy in clothes, but working out will help you look sexy naked.

Dress the Part

Think about how you feel when you go to a party wearing your "million dollar outfit," verses just swinging by in the middle of running errands. Do you feel different? Do you act different? Are you more confident? Social? The same goes with how you dress when you go to the gym, or even when you're working out at home or around the neighborhood.

🍰 Find a few basics that you feel comfortable in at the gym. You don't want to wear your oversized baggy t-shirts with sweat pants and 10-year-old shoes. The nicer and newer the clothes, the more excited you will be to have a chance to wear them! This will encourage you to make the effort.

🍰 Lay your workout clothes out the night before, so they are the first things you see in the morning.

135

🍰 If you plan on working out after work, bring all of your gear with you to work. If you allow yourself to come home first, the couch and TV will start calling your name, and it's <u>so</u> much harder to get moving and back out the door to the gym.

🍰 Invest in a good pair of shoes. It will make all the difference in the world. You may even want to find a specialty store that can test your movement style and actually form a shoe to your foot that will give the least amount of resistance in your movement. They're so much better on your knees, ankles, legs and back.

🍰 Reward yourself with a new piece of workout gear with each small milestone. This will help you build your workout wardrobe, and you will be able to watch the sizes go down with your weight!

Keep It Exciting

To keep yourself from getting bored with the same ol' workout routine each day, find ways to make workouts exciting.

⬢ Set goals that are realistic, and easy for you to keep. Once you're getting into a routine, add to your goals to make them more challenging and possibly more time consuming.

⬢ Keep a playlist of upbeat music. The higher tempo will encourage you to move faster and longer. Music that's 165 to 180 beats per minute is ideal. Search the internet for songs you like in that range.

⬢ Keep updating your playlist as well. New music will keep you on your toes.

⬢ Act like a kid again! Find activities that you used to love as a kid, or activities that your kids love to do, and join them! Running around playing tag is a nice break from the typical treadmill.

🍰 Mix it up. Find different classes and activities that grab your attention.

🍰 Keep up the "extra-curricular" bedroom activities. :)

🍰 Workout with a friend or a group. It's more fun, and you'll be more likely to stick with it.

🍰 Chart your progress! Test yourself when you first start working out to see where you are at. How fast your mile is, how many push-ups you can do, how much weight you can lift. Then re-test yourself every couple of months to see your progress.

🍰 Don't compare yourself to others, compare yourself to the old you and where you came from. People lose weight and burn calories very differently. Men tend to burn 30% to 40% more calories than women do during the same workout due to muscle mass. Keep that in mind if you are being competitive with your partner.

🍰 Strive for excellence, not perfection. No one is perfect, but anyone can be excellent.

🍰 Not a morning person? I can totally relate. If you know you'll never make a 6 AM boot camp, don't sign up for it. You'll just get discouraged every time the snooze button wins the battle. Your workout should be during the time you have the most energy. If that's 2 AM, fantastic! Go with that!

🍰 If you are working out regularly, don't stress over the scale. You may gain some weight in the beginning while your body gains muscle. And since muscle weighs more than fat, this can be frustrating. Instead, measure your fat to muscle ratio. After a while, your body will catch up, your muscle will start burning the fat itself, and all will come full circle on the scale.

Do It Right

🍰 Working out in the morning may save you from making poor decisions the rest of the day. There is something about spending 30 to 45 minutes doing a moderate to vigorous exercise that keeps you from wanting to "ruin" all of your good progress.

🍰 Drink a lot of water!

🍰 Journal all of the exercise and activity you accomplish along side of the food you ate.

🍰 Strength training is just as important as cardio. Muscle burns calories faster than fat does, so the more muscle you have on your body, the less work you have to do to burn calories throughout the day.

🍰 Step it up and join a boot camp. Nothing gets you in shape faster than those intense full-body workouts. If you're limited in funds, they usually cost quite a bit less than personal trainers as well.

🍰 Use hand weights or dumbbells while on the treadmill or while walking around the block. And don't just hold them to your side, use them!

🍰 Invest in a good personal trainer, especially if you're that serious about getting into shape. If you are putting good money into your program, you will be sure to get the most benefits from it. You will also be less likely to skip a workout. It is also a great way to stay accountable. I get that times may be tough, but cut back on things that don't matter instead of cutting back on your health.

🍰 Do the math. Just because you worked out doesn't mean that you have a "free pass" to eat whatever you want. The foods you eat are just as (if not *more*) important than the workouts you do. The point of working out is to increase your weight loss. Not to eat more food.

🍰 Give your self a break. Working out seven days a week is too much. Your body needs time to recover.

🍰 Have a back-up plan for lazy days. If the gym just isn't going to "workout" for you that day, grab your home workout DVD's and equipment that you can use instead. Or just do good 'ol jumping jacks, crunches and push-ups. You'll still feel accomplished even after a quick 30-minute home routine.

🍰 Switch up your routines. If you do the same exact routine for the same amount of time every day, your body will get complacent and used to the workout, and it will stop getting the good benefits from it. Any good trainer will rotate you between different cardio exercises as well as different toning routines. Do the same if you are doing your own routine.

🍰 Sprinting builds more muscle than slow and steady jogging. Try throwing in a few 10 to 60 second sprints into your walk or jog, and then slow down just long enough to catch your breath.

Sneak It In

Find ways to get extra movement in throughout the day. To keep your metabolism moving, <u>you</u> need to keep moving. Some experts say that it's better to do light to moderate activity all day everyday rather than doing an intense workout for one hour, then sitting the rest of the day.

🍰 Park far away from your destination. Walking the distance to do your shopping will help you get those extra steps in throughout the day.

🍰 When bringing shopping bags into the house, bring one bag in at a time. More trips, more movement!

🍰 Use stairs instead of elevators or escalators to burn some extra calories.

🍰 Do a few laps around your office building on your breaks, and after lunch.

🍰 Find easy workouts to do while watching TV. This is much smarter than eating.

🍰 Take a walk around the block, or around your house while talking to your friends on the phone. There is no need to sit while talking.

🍰 Stand more instead of sitting at social get-togethers, and even on the job. The average person burns 100 calories per hour while sitting, and 140 calories per hour while standing.

🍰 Keep weights and workout bands on your coffee table, and use them while catching up on your DVRed TV shows.

🍰 Sit on one of those big exercise balls instead of your couch or computer chair. You'll give your core a mini workout without even thinking about it.

Part 8: Motivation

Losing weight is easy. It takes the same amount of effort to order veggies instead of french fries. The reason why so many people have such a hard time with it is because they don't have the right mindset to keep it up.

The mental side of weight loss is just as important, if not more important, than the knowledge of how to lose weight.

There are several ways to stay motivated, and the truth is, once you're on a roll, it gets easier to just keep going.

Pictures of Yourself and/or Others

Visualizing your success is extremely powerful.

🍰 For some people having an old picture of themselves from back when they were the size they want to be is the most powerful. Others are more motivated by a picture they dislike of themselves at a time when they were at their heaviest. Some are even motivated by a picture of someone else who has their ideal body size. Whatever works for you, have those pictures up in places that will support your good choices.

🍰 If choosing a picture of another person, see if you can Photoshop your face on their body. It's not only fun, but also exciting to see what you will look like in the near future!

🍰 Be creative on where you can keep these pictures. Putting them on the door of your fridge can be powerful. Looking at that picture every time you open the fridge door will help you make better decisions. You could also have pictures in your bathroom, on your dresser, in your car, near your workout equipment, or even by your couch where you are usually lazy.

🍰 You could even keep a photo journal of your weight loss. Take a picture of yourself with each milestone, or maybe each month, and you'll be able to see how fast your efforts are paying off!

Constant Reminders

Find ways to have constant reminders pop up in your everyday life.

🍰 Figure out your "why," write it down, and put it everywhere! In your car, on your closet door, in your wallet, in your kitchen, in your cubicle, everywhere!

🍰 Find healthy apps on your phone that send you reminders to journal your food, or remind you to work out.

🍰 Subscribe to any and every health company's emails you can find. This could include your favorite celebrity trainers, Livestrong™, Weight Watchers®, and even my daily tip!! It's helpful to see these emails in your inbox everyday.

🍰 Subscribe for my daily tips email at www.KaylaWeightLoss.com!

🍰 Set your home screen on your computer to your favorite health site. It could be a daily healthy recipe, or even the site for the weight-loss program you are following. You could even go a step further and set your screen saver to tell you something positive.

🍰 Fill up your DVR with your favorite health shows. A few of my favorites are Extreme Weight Loss, The Biggest Loser®, Dr. Oz, The Doctors, Live Big with Ali Vincent, and other motivational shows.

🍰 Subscribe to health magazines. It will save you so much money to get a monthly subscription than to buy one each month at the store. This way you can subscribe to two or three different magazines, and they will keep showing up at your house.

🍰 Fill your Kindle®, tablet or phone with other healthy books, and make sure that this one is easy to get to as well. ;)

🍰 Write positive messages to yourself on your bathroom mirror with dry erase markers. You could even write on your shower door. There's nothing like waking up to that positive energy, as well as seeing it right before you go to sleep.

Find An Anchor

Find a small token that reminds you to stay on track each day.

🍰 Get a necklace, bracelet, or other piece of jewelry. You may want to reward yourself with one when you hit your first goal. (Which should be something small like your first five or ten pounds.) This will actually give the piece of jewelry a real meaning of weight loss.

🍰 Get a keychain, trinket, or something small like a gratitude rock that you can carry in your pocket. It could even be a lucky coin you've marked with a sticker.

🍰 You could even get something that you hang from your rear-view mirror in your car.

🍰 Make sure that this anchor is specifically a reminder of weight loss, and not a memory attached to something else, like an ex-lover, a parent, or a memory from a vacation you took.

Have Small Goals For Your Milestones

Weight loss is a journey, and the easiest way to hit your destination is to set small goals along the way. Let's just say your goal is to lose 100 pounds. That number can be overwhelming, especially if you're only losing one or two pounds per week (which is a healthy weight loss).

🍰 Set small milestones to hit, and focus on those instead. This could be every five to ten pounds, or it could be losing 5% of your body weight, then 10%, 15%, 20%, etc. It could also be every inch you lose on your waist.

🍰 Try reframing what your goal is. Instead of losing 20 pounds, think of it as losing 1 pound 20 times. It's much easier when you think about it that way.

🍰 Sometimes a visual can help. You could make a glass jar with the amount of stones in it equaling the amount of pounds that you want to lose. With each lost pound, move the stones to another glass jar. If you feel you have an overwhelming amount of weight to lose, do it in phases. Split it up into 2, 3 or 4 amounts, and find a big way to celebrate each jar!

🍰 Have more than one "scale" to track your results. Use measuring tape to keep track the inches you lose, pay attention to how much easier it is to climb the stairs at your office, and notice how much easier it is getting to cross your legs. Your weight scale isn't the only thing that shows how much your efforts are working out for you.

Have Small Goals For Your Behavior

In addition to rewarding yourself with your weight loss, it may be a good idea to find ways to reward yourself with changes in your behavior.

🍰 Each time you say no to not-so-healthy choices, that is a reason to give yourself kudos. It doesn't need to be a big dramatic celebration, but acknowledge the fact that you've grown, and keep it up.

🍰 Maybe you can start a "Kudo's Journal" and keep track of all the great behavior changes you are making along the way.

🍰 Vocalize to your friends and family how much you are growing into this new healthier you. Get them on your side, and also to help you watch your own back if you start to slip.

🍰 Instead of thinking that you "deserve" an unhealthy food, change your thinking and realize that you *really* deserve to be happy, healthy and thin.

🍰 When you feel out of control, think back to a time when it used to be so much worse. We all have our weak moments, but once you start living a healthy lifestyle, your poor choices tend to get better and better. Soon enough, your poor choices will be what you used to call a good choice, and you will see how much you've actually grown.

Your Closet

You look in it everyday. Why not turn it into a piece of motivation?!

🍰 Clean it out!! Go through and get rid of everything you know you will never wear again. You need room for all of the cute new little clothes that will soon be taking over.

🍰 As you go down in sizes, get rid of everything that is too big for you. You don't want a back-up plan of clothes that you can grow back into. If you get rid of it, it will motivate you to keep the pounds off so you don't have to buy bigger clothes ever again.

🍰 You may want to save that one piece of clothing to show you where you came from. Besides, you'll want to be able to take that signature picture of you holding your way-too-big jeans out in front of you when you hit your goal.

🍰 Every once in a while, pick out a dress or an outfit that is just one size too small for you. This will give you motivation to be able to wear it.

🍰 Have a clothes exchange party with some friends. Everyone can bring clothes that are still in good shape, but that either don't fit any longer or maybe you're just not excited about them anymore. Then, you pick out some new favorites and everyone goes home with new exciting clothes for free!

Reward Yourself

Find ways to give kudos to yourself at each milestone. This could be as simple as telling your accountabilibuddy that you hit a goal, or as extravagant as treating yourself to a day at the spa.

🍰 It is suggested that you don't reward yourself with food. You're working on getting away from that habit. When food becomes a reward, it will just affect all of the effort you put into losing weight. If you are looking at using food as a reward, find a healthy but maybe more expensive meal to treat yourself with.

🍰 Pick out a new piece of exercise clothes each time you hit a milestone. You will need it while you lose weight anyway, and it's a great positive reinforcement.

🍰 If money is tight, treat yourself to a spa day at home! Light some candles, soak in a bubble bath, read your favorite book, give yourself a hot oil treatment, and give your feetsies a foot mask and scrub. Ahhhh…. Heaven at home!

🍰 Some other rewards may be-

- A mani-pedi

- A new book, DVD, or album

- Clothes and shoes

- A movie or a play

- Going to a sports game

- New bedding

- New flowers for your garden

- Hiring a personal trainer

- A new phone or other electronic device

🍰 Start a collection of things you enjoy, like candles or trinkets of some sort. You can get a new one with each milestone or pound lost. These will also serve as a great anchor.

🍰 Create a reward chart! For each of your major milestones, specify the bigger rewards you want to treat yourself to. Have fun crossing off each pound you lose while you get closer and closer to your rewards!

🍰 It may be a good idea to have a grand reward for when you hit your ultimate goal. It will really give you something to look forward to and to work towards! Maybe it's a good time to upgrade to a new car, or go on that vacation you keep talking about.

🍰 Another fantastic idea is to start saving up for that brand new wardrobe you know you're going to need! For each pound you lose, or for each week you are on plan, set aside a certain amount of money that will add up for your shopping spree. You could even complete that with a full makeover! There's nothing like showing off the "new you," in such a fashionable and exciting way.

Part 9: Staying In Control

Now that you have all of the information you need to make smart decisions, it's time to make sure you have everything you need to stay motivated and in control.

A coach, a trainer, a friend, a support system, and a plan are all things that can help you stay in control, and on the right path to hit your goals.

How serious are you about keeping your weight off once you hit your goal? Outside support might be just what you need.

Find Support

The easiest way to stay on track is to have a support system. And the only way to get a support system is to talk about what your plans are.

🍰 Tell your friends and family that you are working on getting healthy. Make sure that you are talking about it in a positive way. If you're moping around complaining about all the foods that you "can't eat" your family is going to naturally want to make you happy, and they think that pushing fatty foods in your face will make you happy.

🍰 Instead, focus on being positive in the way you talk. Let them know that you are excited about losing weight and getting healthy, and that you would like their support. Most likely there will be people in your life who are looking for a support system to help them get started as well. Step up and show them all of the great things you have learned!

🍰 Find an accountabilibuddy! Find someone who will keep you accountable and call you out when you need it. They should be positive, but not too soft on you. They should be excited in the direction you are going, and not someone is will eventually try to pull you back. Try to find someone who is a great example of your ultimate goal.

🍰 Be careful of people who may get jealous. It's sad, but there may be people who feel threatened by your success. Don't let these people get you down. You are 100% worth the effort you are putting in to your plan. Instead, try to find people who are supportive to spend your time around.

🍰 Start a blog, and focus it on your goal and your accomplishments. It's harder to quit in front of an audience.

🍰 Get a coach! I'm available for personal, one-on-one sessions, either via phone or Skype, and for group coaching. Visit www.KaylaWeightLoss.com for info.

Create A Calendar

Planning ahead makes the biggest difference with weight loss. Remember, if you fail to plan, then you're planning to fail.

🍰 Each week you should look at what activities are coming up. If you are on a plan that allows flexibility, decide which days you plan on splurging a bit, and which days you plan to keep super healthy. This way, it's easier to not slip up and run out of options when it comes to important parties, and events.

🍰 You should also mark which days you will fit in time for exercise and activities. You'll want to be specific with certain times and activities that you plan on doing, too. It may be harder to keep it up if it's not a solid plan in your calendar.

🍰 You'll also want to pick a specific day for your shopping and prepping. Especially when you're first starting out, you may spend a bit more time at the grocery store making your smart decisions. Then you'll want to make sure you have time to come home to clean and prep all of your fruits and vegetables so they are ready to go for the week.

Invest In A Coach

Many people believe that the reason why they can't lose weight is because of their diet, their lack of time, their medical issues, the fact they eat out too often, or because of their genes. I know this because I used to be one of those people. The truth is that the biggest part of weight loss is your mindset. And that is where a coach comes into the picture.

A coach will keep you accountable, and at cause for your decisions.

A good coach will help you see things outside of your box. They know that there is always a solution, so they will help you come up with one for each of your situations you may run into.

Your own decisions and limiting beliefs can sabotage you, and a coach will help you keep a positive mindset, and power in the belief that you can accomplish anything and everything you start.

🍰 Coaching people through weight loss is my specialty. Check out my website at www.kaylaweightloss.com to set up a consultation and I'll show you just how easy and fun eliminating those extra pounds can be!

About the Author

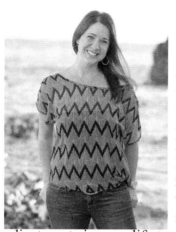

Kayla Moffett is an author, speaker and weight loss coach in Newport Beach, CA.

After struggling with her own weight for years, she finally cracked the code and lost over 70 pounds. More importantly, she learned to keep it off. She now teaches others how to use easy tips, tricks and strategies to make simple adjustments in your life to get the body you desire.

You can find out more about Kayla and sign up for her daily tips email newsletter at:

www.KaylaWeightLoss.com

4715560R00093

Made in the USA
San Bernardino, CA
02 October 2013